Ultimate Partner Workouts

Increase Fitness Level and Quality Time Together With These Fun Couple Exercises

RON KNESS

Contents

Disclaimer

All information is intended for your general knowledge only and is not a substitute for medical advice or treatment. You should seek medical advice before starting this or any other weight loss or fitness regimen. We make no warranty, express or implied, regarding your individual results.

The author disclaims any personal liability, for loss or risk incurred as a result of any information or advice contained herein, either directly or indirectly.

All links are for informational purposes only and are not warranted for content, accuracy, or other implied or explicit purposes. All links were working at the time of this eBook's release but may now have expired.

The author does not intend to render legal, accounting or other professional advice in the documents contained herein. The reader is encouraged to seek competent legal and accounting advice before engaging in any business activity.

This eBook may not be sold or given away. Unauthorized distribution, resell, or copying of this material is unlawful. The author reserves the right to use the full force of the law in the protection of its intellectual property including the contents, ideas, and expressions contained herein.

See your healthcare professional before starting any diet, health or exercise program!

Introduction

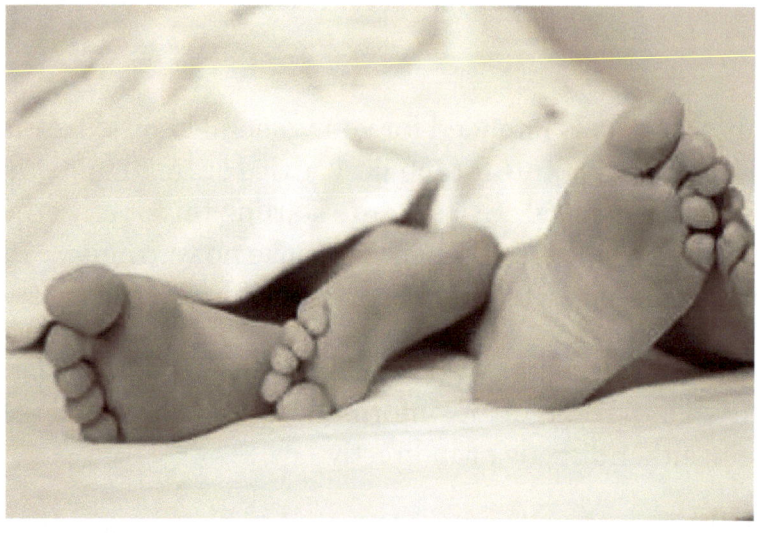

Working out regularly has many benefits. It improves your cardiovascular fitness, keeps all your major organs healthy, protects you from disease, boosts your immune system and much more.

Unfortunately, if you're in a relationship, it also eats into one of your most valuable commodities – quality time with your partner. For example, if you work out five times a week, have a full-time job and have commitments at the weekend, there's very little time left to see your partner and spend time with them.

The good news is that there is a solution to this problem – Partner Workouts. By performing partner workouts, you can spend extra time with your partner and achieve your fitness goals at the same time. Partner workouts also have numerous other benefits which include:

Improved Sex Life: Regular workouts improve your strength, stamina and flexibility which are all good attributes to have in the bedroom and can greatly improve your sex life. In addition to this, toning up your muscles and reducing your body fat levels helps you look more attractive to your partner which ultimately makes sex more enjoyable for both of you. Who couldn't use more time between the sheets!

Motivation: Working out together allows you to keep each other motivated. If you're having a bad day and don't feel like working out, your partner can inspire you to workout. Likewise, if your partner doesn't feel like working out, you can motivate them to power through and fit in a workout.

Shared Interest: One of the biggest problems in relationships is that as time passes, you have less and less activities that you do as a couple which means less shared interests and less things to talk about. With partner workouts, you can develop a very strong shared interest that brings you together on an almost daily basis, along with improving both of your fitness levels.

Stronger Relationship: As well as giving you and your partner a powerful shared interest, partner workouts also strengthen your relationship in other ways. For example, the extra time you spend together, gives you more opportunities to talk. Working out together also gives you plenty of opportunities to complement each other on the way you look or congratulate each other for achieving fitness goals.

In this book, I'm going to help you formulate your partner workouts by providing you with a list 30 partner exercises that you can do together as a couple.

As with all types of exercise, make sure you start off slowly when trying these partner exercises for the first time and slowly increase the pace once you get used to the movements.

NOTE: In exercises where a piece or two of equipment are recommended, it is listed in the Resources Chapter with a link to a suggested piece. If you buy through that link, I get a small commission from each sale.

Balance Exercises

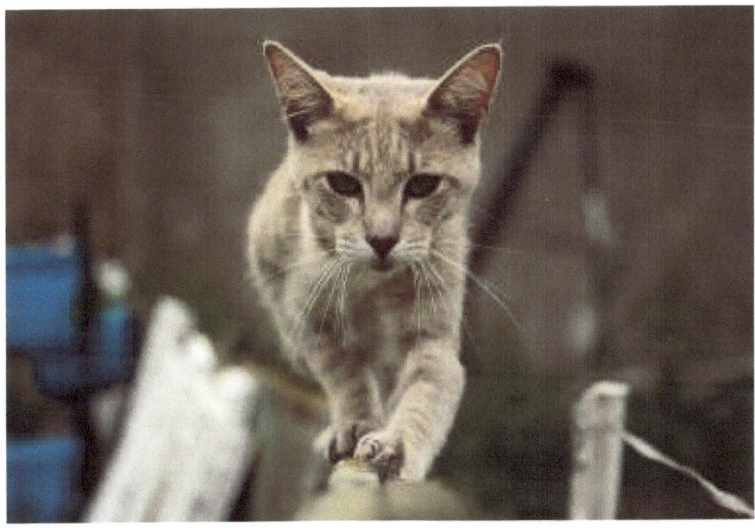

Good balance is essential for almost every type of exercise. Not only do these partner exercises help improve your balance but they're also incredibly fun. In fact, most of the exercises play out more like games than exercises and encourage friendly competition between you and your partner.

1. Back-To-Back Partner Stand-Ups

Equipment Required:
None.

Instructions:
Sit back-to-back with your partner with your knees bent as far as possible and your feet planted firmly on the floor. Hook your arms together and then slowly stand up by straightening your legs and pushing against each other's backs.

Once you've managed to stand up, slowly lower yourselves back down to the starting position. Repeat as many times as you desire.

Back-To-Back Partner Stand-Up Variations:
Once you've mastered the basics of back-to-back partner stand ups, give the variations below a try and make it even more challenging:

- *Perform back-to-back partner stand ups using just one leg each (this variation is very difficult, so only attempt it if you and your partner both have very good balance skills).*

- *Perform back-to-back partner stand ups while holding light dumbbells in your hands. This will strengthen your leg muscles at the same time as improving your balance.*

2. BOSU Tug-Of-War

Equipment Required:
2 BOSU balls.
2 resistance bands.

Instructions:
Place the two BOSU balls on the floor with the dome sides facing up and make sure they are far enough apart so that the resistance bands will be fully extended when stretched between them.

Grab a handle of one resistance band with your left hand and one resistance band with your right hand and get your partner to do the same.

Stand on one of the BOSU balls, get your balance and bend your knees. Get your partner stand on the other BOSU ball and do the same.

Hold the resistance bands above your head, get your partner to do the same and then stretch the resistance bands until they are tight.

When you are both ready and in position, start pulling the resistance bands and try to pull each other off the BOSU balls.

Once one partner has successfully pulled the other partner off the BOSU ball, they gain a point.

Create a scoring system (either first person to x number of points or the best of x rounds) and then play until you have a winner.

BOSU Tug-Of-War Variations:
When you've played BOSU tug of war a few times, try the variations below to make it even more difficult:

- *Flip the BOSU balls so that the platform sides are up and then perform the exercise as normal. The platform side is much less stable than the dome side and will provide you with an even greater balance challenge.*

- *Wear ankle and wrist weights while playing BOSU tug of war. This will help build up your strength at the same time as your balance because you will be carrying more weight and need to use more force to pull your partner off the BOSU ball.*

3. Single Leg Balance With Partner

Equipment Required:
None.

Instructions:
Stand face-to-face with your partner about an arm's width apart. Bring your right foot off the ground, balance on your left leg and get your partner to do the same.

Bend your right knee and your hips slightly and get your partner to do the same.

When you are both balanced and ready, take turns at pushing each other off balance.

Once one partner has successful pushed the other partner off balance (by making them put their right foot on the ground), they gain a point.

Create a scoring system (either first person to x number of points or the best of x rounds) and then play until you have a winner. Once you have a winner, repeat steps 1 to 6 but balance on your right leg instead of your left leg.

Single Leg Balance With Partner Variations:

The single leg balance with partner exercise is very challenging at first but once you've had a bit of practice, you may want to spice it up. To do this, give one of the variations below a try:

- *Get your partner to stand on two legs and try to push you off balance while you are on one leg. Once you lose your balance, switch and get them to stand on one leg as you try to push them off balance while standing on both legs. The winner is the one who stays balanced for longest.*

- *Wear ankle and wrist weights while practicing the single leg balance with partner exercise. This will help build up your strength at the same time as your balance because you will be carrying more weight and need to use more force to knock your partner off balance.*

4. Single Leg BOSU Catch

Equipment Required:
2 BOSU balls.
1 small medicine ball.

Instructions:
Place the two BOSU balls on the floor with the dome side facing up about five feet apart. Grab the medicine ball, stand on one of the BOSU balls, raise your left leg and get your balance on your right leg. Get your partner to balance on their right leg on the other BOSU ball.

Throw the medicine ball to your partner and get them to catch it while remaining balanced on your right leg at all times. Get them to throw the medicine ball back to you and then continue tossing it back and forth, making sure that you both stay balanced on your right legs at all times.

The first person to drop the medicine ball or lose their balance loses and this gives the other partner a point.

Create a scoring system (either first person to x number of points or the best of x rounds) and then play until you have a winner. Once you have a winner, repeat steps 1 to 6 but balance on your left leg instead of your right leg.

Single Leg BOSU Catch Variations:

The single BOSU catch does take some time to get used to. However, once you've mastered it, give the following variations a try:

- *Get your partner to stand on two legs and throw the medicine ball to you at various heights and angles while you stand on the BOSU ball with one leg. Once you lose your balance, switch and get them to stand on the BOSU ball with one leg as you throw the BOSU ball to them while standing on both legs. The winner is the one who stays balanced for longest.*

- *Flip the BOSU balls so that the platform sides are up and then perform the exercise as normal. The platform side is much less stable than the dome side and will test your balance to a greater degree.*

5. Single Leg Partner Jump Shadow

Equipment Required:
None.

Instructions:
Stand face to face with your partner about two feet apart. Bring your right foot off the ground and balance on your left leg.
Get your partner to bring their left foot off the ground and balance on their right leg.

Pick one partner to be the offensive person and the other partner to be the defensive person. The offensive person is responsible for initiating movements and can hop to the left, right, forwards or backwards.

The defensive person has to mimic the offensive person's movements as quickly as possible.

Start hopping and continue until one partner loses their balance. Once this happens, the partner who stayed balanced gets a point.

Create a scoring system (either first person to x number of points or the best of x rounds) and then play until you have a winner. Once you have a winner, repeat steps 1 to 7 but switch the legs you are balancing on.

Single Leg Partner Jump Shadow Variations:
Once your balance improves and you can do the single leg partner jump shadow exercise without falling over for long periods of time, try the variations below to make it more challenging:

- *Get the offensive person to stand still and shout fast paced instructions to the defensive person. The winner is the defensive person who stays balanced for the longest.*

- *Wear ankle and wrist weights while performing the single leg partner jump shadow exercise. This will help build up your strength at the same time as your balance because you will be carrying more weight and need to use more force to hop in the various directions.*

Bodyweight Exercises

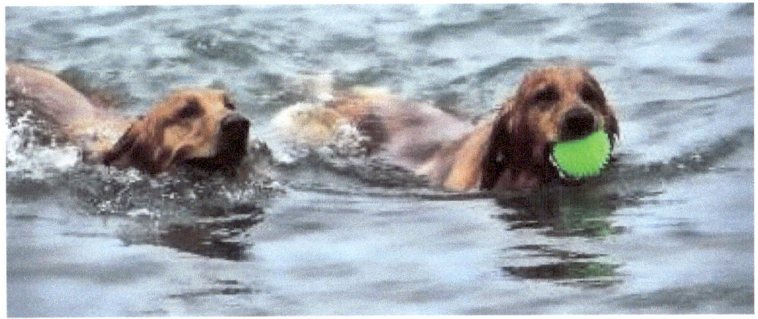

Bodyweight exercises are simple and require no equipment. These partner bodyweight exercises are also extremely more fun as they allow you to interact with each other while you exercise and prevent boredom from setting in.

1. Bodyweight Partner Lunges

Equipment Required:
1 resistance band.

Instructions:
Stand face to face with your partner, holding one side of the resistance band each and step back until it's tight. Once the resistance band is tight, step back with your left foot and get your partner to do the same.

Bend your knees and slowly lower your bodies down until your knees are at a 90-degree angle, making sure that they don't go over your ankles.

Slowly raise your bodies back up to the starting position. Step forward with your left foot, then step back with your right foot and get your partner to do the same.

Bend your knees and slowly lower your bodies down until your knees are at a 90-degree angle, making sure that they don't go over your ankles.

Slowly raise your bodies back up to the starting position. Repeat for as many repetitions as you desire.

Bodyweight Partner Lunges Variations:
Once you get used to the technique and find your balance, you'll be able to perform bodyweight partner lunges with ease. To mix them up and keep them challenging, try the suggestions below:

- *Instead of holding a resistance, grab each other's forearms to lunge from a different angle and target different leg muscles.*

- *Wear a weighted vest while performing bodyweight partner lunges. This will give your leg muscles an even better workout as you will be pushing up more weight as you lunge.*

2. Bodyweight Partner Squats

Equipment Required:
1 rope.

Instructions:
Stand face to face with your partner about an arm's width apart. Grab the rope with your both hands and get your partner to do the same, leaving a small gap between your two pairs of hands.

Slowly bend your legs and lower your bodies down until both your butts are parallel with your knees.

Slowly straighten your legs and raise your bodies back up to the starting position. Repeat for as many repetitions as you desire.

Bodyweight Partner Squats Variations:
Bodyweight partner squats are difficult initially but with a little practice, you'll get used to the technique. Once you're well practiced, try out the following variations to keep the exercise fresh:

- *Instead of holding a rope, grab each other's forearms to squat from a different angle and target different leg muscles.*

- *Perform bodyweight partner squats using just one leg each (this variation is very difficult, so only attempt it if you and your partner both have very good balance skills).*

3. Partner Planks With Clap

Equipment Required:
None.

Instructions:
Kneel down and place your forearms on the floor in front of you. Get your partner to place their forearms on the floor in the same way and ensure that they are about an arms width away from you.

Straighten your legs out behind you, tighten up your core muscles and balance on your toes and forearms. Get your partner to do the same. Hold this plank position and then both slowly raise your right elbows off the floor, reach forward and clap your right hands together.

Put your right elbows back on the floor and then slowly raise your left elbows off the floor, reach forward and clap your left hands together.
Continue clapping your right and left hands together as described above and hold the plank for as long as you can.

Partner Planks With Clap Variations:
Once you've perfected your partner plank with clap form, check out the variations below to make this exercise even tougher:

- *Instead of clapping your hands together, reach right across and tap each other's shoulders. Doing this will make you stretch further and boost your balance and core strength to a greater degree.*

- *Wear a weighted vest while performing the partner planks with clap exercise. This will give your core strength an even greater boost as you will be supporting more weight during the plank.*

4. Partner Push Ups With Clap

Equipment Required:
None.

Instructions:

Place your hands on the floor and make sure they are parallel to your chest. Get your partner to place their hands on the floor in the same way and ensure that they are about an arms width away from you.

Straighten your legs out behind you and tighten up your core muscles. Get your partner to do the same.

Once you are both ready, slowly bend your arms at the same time and lower your bodies down until your noses touch the floor.

Once your noses touch the floor, slowly straighten your arms and return to the starting position.

Reach out towards each other with your right hands and clap them together. Put your right hands back on the floor and then repeat steps 3 and 4.

Reach out towards each other with your left hands and clap them together. Put your left hands back on the floor and then repeat steps 3 to 7 for as many repetitions as you desire.

Partner Push Ups With Clap Variations:

After you've mastered these partner push ups with clap, give the suggestions below a try to increase the difficulty level:

- *Instead of clapping your hands together straight away, tuck your legs in after each push up, jump up and then clap your hands together. Doing this brings your legs into play and gives you a full body workout.*

- *Wear a weighted vest while performing the partner push-ups with clap exercise. This will help build up your strength even further as you will be pushing up more weight with every rep.*

5. Partner Wheelbarrow

Equipment Required:
None.

Instructions:
Find a space where you can take between 10 and 20 steps without anyone blocking your path.
Stand in front of your partner, place your hands on the ground and get your partner to hold your legs.

Keep your core muscles tight and start walking forward with your hands. Get your partner to follow behind you at the same pace.

Complete two laps of your workout space and then get your partner to put your legs back on the ground. Switch positions so that you are standing behind your partner. Get them to place their hands on the ground and hold their legs. Walk forward and get them to walk forward with their hands at the same pace.

Complete two laps of your workout space and then put your partner's legs on the ground. Repeat as many times as you desire.

Partner Wheelbarrow Variations:

There are many ways that you can increase the intensity of partner wheelbarrows. Once you've got used to the exercise, try out the variations below:

- *Turn your fingers inwards when walking on your hands to further enhance your core stability.*

- *Instead of walking on your hands, bend your arms and hop forward while in the wheelbarrow position. This will target your chest and arms and give you a fantastic upper body workout.*

- *Wear a weighted vest while walking on your hands. This will help build up your core strength even further as you will be supporting a greater amount of weight as you move.*

Flexibility Exercises

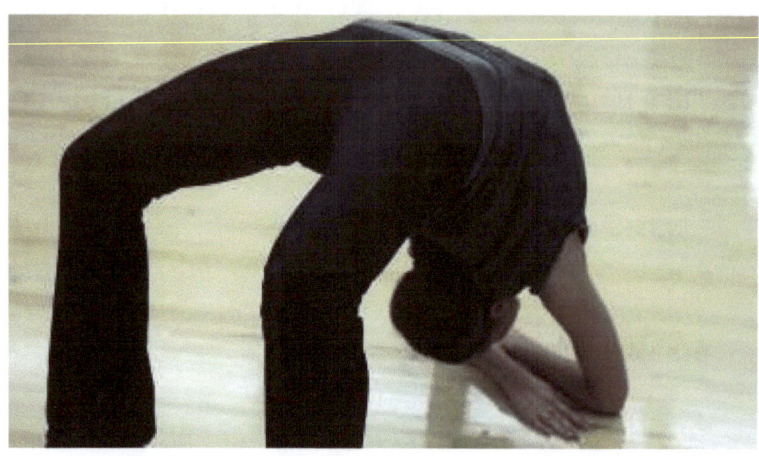

Good flexibility increases your range of motion, reduces your chance of injury and makes exercising much easier. It also enhances your day to day life and can make many common aches and pains disappear. These partner flexibility exercises are a great way to get maximum results from your flexibility training, as very often having a partner present can help you stretch that little bit further.

1. Back-To-Back Stretch

Equipment Required:
None.

Instructions:
Sit back-to-back with your partner and cross both of your legs. Stretch forward as far as you can go and get your partner to lean backwards to hold you in position.

Hold the stretch for 30 seconds. After 30 seconds, slowly lean backwards and get your partner to lean forward as far as they can go. Hold the stretch for 30 seconds.

Partner Back To Back Stretch Variations:
Once you've practiced the partner back-to-back stretch for a few weeks and your back has become more supple, give the variations below a try to keep the exercise interesting:

- *Instead of sitting opposite each other, get one partner to stretch forward and one partner to stand behind them and gently push them into the stretch. Hold the position for 30 seconds, swap and then repeat the stretch with the other partner.*

- *Straighten your legs and perform the stretch as above to place greater focus on your legs and further improve their flexibility.*

2. Partner Lying Hamstring Stretch

Equipment Required:
None.

Instructions:
Lie on your back and raise your right leg into the air, making sure to keep it straight. Get your partner to stand to the side of your leg and stretch it back as far as it will go.

Hold it in position for 30 seconds. After 30 seconds, get your partner to slowly lower your leg back down to the floor.

Get your partner to lie down on the floor and raise their right leg into the air, making sure to keep it straight. Stand by the side of their leg and stretch it as far back as it will go.

Hold it in position for 30 seconds. After 30 seconds, slowly lower your partner's leg back down to the floor.

Repeat steps 1 to 8 using your left legs instead of your right legs.

Partner Lying Hamstring Stretch Variations:
After a few weeks of performing the partner lying hamstring stretch, your flexibility should improve quite significantly. Once your flexibility does improve, try the variations below to keep the exercise challenging:

- *Get your partner to stretch your leg back as far as it can go and hold it in position for 30 seconds as described above.*

- *After 30 seconds, keep trying to hold the stretch as your partner attempts to push your leg towards the floor. Swap and repeat the stretch with your partner. This extra resistance at the end of the exercise will boost your flexibility, core strength and leg strength.*

- *Wear ankle weights while performing the partner lying hamstring stretch. This will help build up your leg strength and core strength at the same time as your flexibility and give you a great lower body workout.*

3. Partner Open Leg Stretch

Equipment Required:
None.

Instructions:

Sit opposite your partner, open out your legs while keeping them straight and put your feet together. Reach out and grab each other's hands.

Get your partner to slowly pull backwards as you stretch forward as far as you can go. Once you are stretched as forward as you can go, tell your partner to hold you in that position for 30 seconds.

After 30 seconds, slowly raise yourself back up and then pull backwards and get your partner to stretch forward.

Once they are stretched as far forward as they can go, hold the position for 30 seconds. After 30 seconds, slowly raise yourself back up to the starting position.

Partner Leg Stretch Variations:

If you want to add a bit of variety to your partner open leg stretches, try the alternative versions of this exercise below:

- *Close your legs and perform the stretch as above to place greater focus on your legs and further improve their flexibility.*

- *Instead of sitting opposite each other, get one partner to stretch and one partner to stand behind them and gently ease them into the stretch. Hold the position for 30 seconds, swap and then repeat the stretch with the other partner.*

4. Partner Shoulder Stretch

Equipment Required:
None.

Instructions:
Hold your arms out straight to the side with the palms of your hands facing the floor. Get your partner to stand behind you and gently pull your arms backwards until your shoulder blades are stretched out as far as you can go.

Hold the stretch for 30 seconds. After 30 seconds, get your partner to release your arms and switch positions.

Get them to hold their arms out straight to the side with the palms of their hands facing the floor. Gently pull their arms backwards until their shoulder blades are stretched out as far as they can go.

Hold that position for 30 seconds. After 30 seconds, release their arms.

Partner Shoulder Stretch Variations:
After you've gained some flexibility in your shoulders, try the following variations to keep partner shoulder stretches fresh and exciting:

- *Get your partner to stretch your shoulders back as far as they will go and hold them in that position for 30 seconds as described above. After 30 seconds, keep trying to hold the stretch as your partner attempts to push your arms forward. This extra resistance at the end of the exercise will boost your shoulder strength along with your flexibility.*

- *Perform partner shoulder stretches while holding light dumbbells in your hands. This will strengthen your shoulders and enhance their flexibility at the same time.*

5. Partner Tricep Stretch

Equipment Required:
None.
Instructions:
Raise your left arm and bend it behind your neck. Get your partner to stand behind you and gently pull your left hand down your back as far as it will go.

Hold the stretch for 30 seconds. After 30 seconds, get your partner to release your left arm, raise your right arm and bend it behind your neck.

Get your partner to gently pull your right hand down your back as far as it will go. Hold the stretch for 30 seconds.

Switch positions and repeat steps 1 to 6 with your partner stretching and you assisting.

Partner Tricep Stretch Variations:
In the early stages, your triceps are naturally inflexible. However, once you've practiced this exercise a few times and increased their flexibility, give the alternatives below a try to make your tricep stretches even more challenging:

- *Instead of getting the partner assisting the stretch to pull down on the hands of the partner who is stretching, get them to gently push down on their elbows. This places greater emphasis on the shoulder and helps improve your flexibility in this area.*

- *Wear wrist weights while performing the partner tricep stretch to boost your arm strength along with your flexibility.*

Medicine Ball Exercises

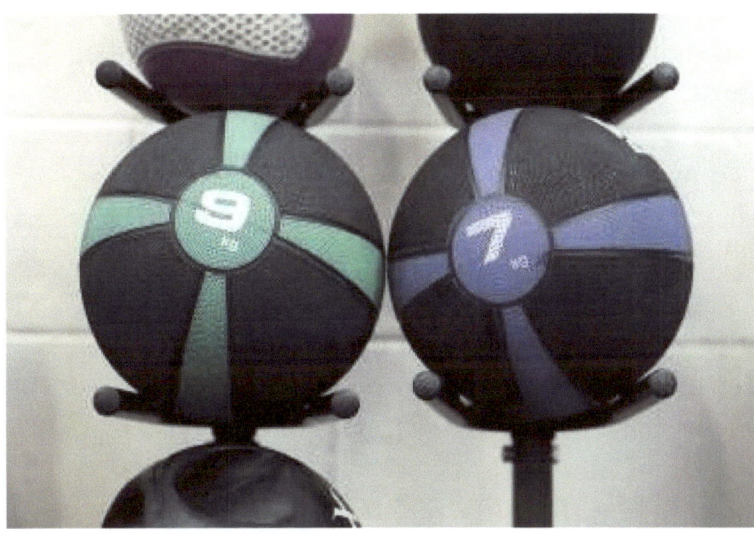

The medicine ball is a brilliant piece of exercise equipment that can be used to enhance your balance, reflexes and strength. These partner medicine ball workouts are highly enjoyable and in most cases, they work your entire body.

1. Medicine Ball Chest Pass

Equipment Required:
1 small medicine ball.

Instructions:
Stand about 10 feet away from your partner and make sure you are facing each other. Grab the medicine ball in both of your hands, bend your elbows and bring it towards your chest.

Bend your knees and slowly lower your body down until your knees are at a 90-degree angle, making sure that they don't go over your ankles. Straighten your knees and as you come up, straighten your arms and throw the medicine ball towards your partner.

Get your partner to repeat steps 2 to 4 and throw the medicine ball back to you. Repeat for as many repetitions as you desire.

Medicine Ball Chest Pass Variations:
Once you and your partner have become pros at the medicine ball chest pass, try mixing the exercise up a little with the variations below:
- *Jump in the air as you throw the medicine ball to each other to further target your leg muscles.*

- *Wear ankle and wrist weights while performing medicine ball chest passes to build additional strength in your upper and lower body.*

2. Medicine Ball Partner Slams

Equipment Required:
1 small medicine ball.

Instructions:
Stand about 10 feet away from your partner and make sure you are facing each other. Grab the medicine ball in both of your hands and hold it above your head.

Slam the medicine ball down in the middle of the space between you and your partner, so that it bounces into their hands.

Get your partner to catch the medicine ball and then slam it down in the middle of the space between you and your partner, so that it bounces into your hands. Repeat for as many repetitions as you desire.

Medicine Ball Partner Slams Variations:
Medicine ball partner slams are an excellent upper body exercise that really work your arms, shoulders and chest. However, if you want to increase the intensity, try the following variations:

- *Instead of facing each other, stand back to back then twist and slam the medicine ball to each other, alternating between your left and right sides.*

- *Wear wrist weights while performing medicine ball partner slams to add even more upper body resistance and further enhance the strength of your arms, chest and shoulders.*

3. Medicine Ball Partner Twists

Equipment Required:
1 small medicine ball.

Instructions:
Sit to the side of your partner and make sure you are about 5 feet apart. Bend your knees, lean back slightly, take your feet off the floor and tighten your core muscles. Get your partner to do the same.

Grab the medicine ball with both hands and twist it to the right, to the left, back to the right and then throw it to your partner.

Instruct your partner to twist the medicine ball to the left, to the right, to the left and then throw it back to you. Repeat for as many repetitions as you desire.

Medicine Ball Partner Twists Variations:
Medicine ball partner twists give your core a fantastic workout. However, if you want to make them more difficult, give the following alternative versions of this exercise a try:

- *Instead of sitting up while performing medicine ball partner twists, lie flat on your back to place more focus on your upper body and strengthen your arms, chest and shoulders.*

- *Instead of sitting up while performing medicine ball partner twists, stand up straight to target your core in a different way.*

4. Medicine Ball Sit Up & Pass

Equipment Required:
1 small medicine ball.

Instructions:
Sit opposite your partner and hook your ankles together. Grab the medicine ball and hold it against your chest.

Lie back, raise the medicine ball above your head and touch it against the floor behind you. Sit up and pass the medicine ball to your partner.

Get your partner to lie back, raise the medicine ball above their head and touch it against the floor behind them.

Get your partner to sit up and pass the medicine ball back to you. Repeat for as many repetitions as you desire.

Medicine Ball Sit Up & Pass Variations:
The medicine ball sit up and pass is a very challenging exercise. However, once you master it, try the following variations to make it even more intense:

- *Instead of passing the medicine ball to your partner, throw it to them from behind your head while you are lying down. This brings your arms, chest and shoulders into play and helps to strengthen them.*

- *Instead of sitting opposite each other, get one partner to stand about 10 feet away from the other partner and throw the medicine ball to them as they perform sit ups and pass it back. Perform as many repetitions as you like, then swap and repeat the exercise.*

5. Medicine Ball Unders & Overs

Equipment Required:
1 small medicine ball.

Instructions:
Stand back to back with your partner and hold the medicine ball in both hands. Lift the medicine ball above your head and pass it to your partner.

Get your partner to drop down and pass the medicine ball to you through their legs.

Bend over, grab the medicine ball and then stand back up, lift the medicine ball above your head and pass it to your partner. Repeat for as many repetitions as you desire.

Medicine Ball Unders & Overs Variations:
Medicine ball unders and overs are an excellent full body workout. However, if you want to make them more difficult, give the variations below a try:

- *Randomly change direction when performing medicine ball unders and overs to test you and your partner's reflexes.*

- *Wear ankle and wrist weights while performing medicine ball unders and overs to add extra resistance and boost your overall strength.*

Free Weight Exercises

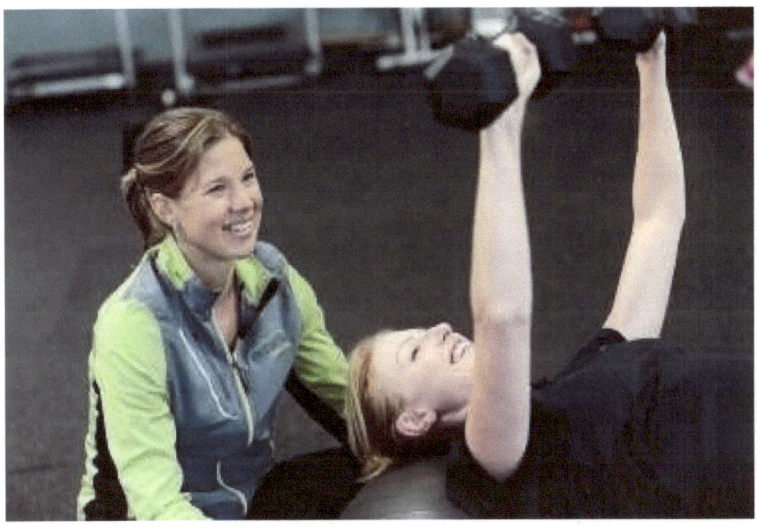

Free weights are a fantastic way to build up the muscles in all parts of your body. These partner exercises allow you to add extra variety to your free weight routines and in doing so keep them fresh and exciting.

1. Negative Bicep Dumbbell Curls

Equipment Required:
2 dumbbells.

Instructions:
Grab the dumbbells, hold them down by your side and stand face to face with your partner. Get your partner to lift the dumbbells for you until your arms are fully curled and then get them to take a step back.

Slowly lower the dumbbells back to the starting position and maintain full tension in your biceps as you lower them.

Repeat steps 2 and 3 for as many repetitions as you desire.

Hand the dumbbells to your partner and lift the dumbbells for them until their arms are fully curled, then take a step back. Get your partner to slowly lower the dumbbells back to the starting position and maintain full tension in their biceps as they lower them.

Repeat steps 5 and 6 for as many repetitions as they desire.

Negative Bicep Dumbbell Curls Variations:
Once you've mastered the form required for negative bicep curls, give these alternative versions of the exercise a try to make it even more challenging:

- *Get the partner who is supporting the curl to push upwards against the hands of the partner performing the exercise during the negative part of the curl. This provides extra resistance and helps to further tone your biceps.*

- *Swap the dumbbells for kettlebells to challenge your biceps in a slightly different way.*

2. Partner Barbell Deadlifts

Equipment Required:
1 barbell.

Instructions:
Stand next to your partner in front of the barbell. Bend over, bend your knees slightly and place your hands on the barbell.

Slowly straighten your backs and your knees and lift the barbell off the ground as you do.

Slowly return to the starting position and lower the barbell back onto the floor. Repeat for as many repetitions as you desire.

Partner Barbell Deadlifts Variations:
Once you've mastered the basic partner deadlift, give the variations below a try to further increase the intensity:

- *After each deadlift, drop down and do a sit-up. This will target your core along with your legs.*

- *After each deadlift, keep hold of the barbell, kick out your legs behind you and perform a burpee. This allows you to add a cardiovascular element to the exercise and burn more calories.*

3. Partner Barbell Sit-Ups

Equipment Required:
1 barbell.

Instructions:
Sit down next to your partner with your knees bent, your feet planted flat on the floor and hold a barbell between the two of you. Slowly lie back and then sit back up while keeping the barbell held against your chests. Repeat for as many repetitions as you desire.

Partner Barbell Sit Ups Variations:
Partner barbell sit ups are a fantastic way to tighten up your core muscles and get washboard abs. However, once you've practiced them for a while and need a bit more of a challenge, give the following variations a try:

- *After each sit up, stand up, curl the barbell, then drop back down and repeat. This will strengthen your arms along with your core.*

- *After each sit up, stand up, press the barbell above your heads, then drop back down and repeat. This will strengthen your shoulders along with your core.*

4. Partner Kettlebell Swings

Equipment Required:
1 kettlebell.

Instructions:
Grab the kettlebell and stand about 5 feet away from your partner, making sure you are facing each other. Place the kettlebell on the ground, in between your legs and just in front of your feet.

Bend your knees, reach down and pick the kettlebell up and then swing it upwards, straighten your knees and throw it towards your partner.

Get your partner to catch it, bend their knees, swing the kettlebell between their legs and then swing it upwards, straighten their knees and throw it back to you. Repeat for as many repetitions as you desire.

Partner Kettlebell Swings Variations:
After you've had some practice with partner kettlebell swings, give the alternative versions below a try and make it even more challenging:

- *Instead of swinging a kettlebell, swing a dumbbell to target your muscles in a slightly different way.*

- *Instead of swinging the kettlebell in a straight line from between your legs, swing the kettlebell from left to target different muscle groups.*

5. *Superman Dumbbell Pass*

Equipment Required:
2 stability balls.
1 dumbbell.

Instructions:
Place the stability balls on the floor about 5 feet apart. Grab one end of the dumbbell in each hand and kneel down in front of your stability ball. Get your partner to kneel in front of their stability ball.

Lean forward, rest your stomach on the stability ball, stretch your legs out behind you and get your balance. Get your partner to adopt the same position on their stability ball. Hold your hands out in front of you and get your partner to do the same. Pass the dumbbell to your partner.

Get them to rotate their arms backwards while keeping their balance on the stability ball and holding the dumbbell in their right hand. While their arms are behind their back, get them to pass the dumbbell from their right hand to their left hand and then bring their arms forward.

Get them to pass the dumbbell to you. Rotate your arms backwards while keeping your balance on the stability ball and holding the dumbbell in your right hand.

While your arms are behind your back, pass the dumbbell from your right hand to your left hand and then bring your arms forward. Repeat steps 5 to 10 for as many repetitions as you desire.

Superman Dumbbell Pass Variations:
The superman dumbbell pass is an extremely challenging exercise that tests your balance, core strength and stability. However, once you have mastered it, try the following variations to keep it fresh and exciting:

- *Instead of using a stability ball, perform superman dumbbell passes on a BOSU ball for a different type of balance challenge.*

- *Wear wrist weights while performing superman dumbbell passes to build up even more strength in your arms.*

Cardio Exercises

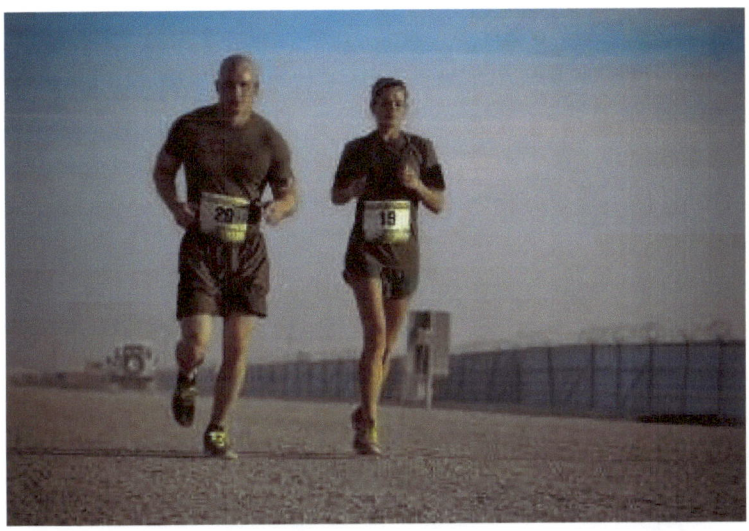

Having a good level of cardiovascular fitness boost your stamina, improves your mood, protects you from a range of chronic disease and much more. However, many people find traditional cardio exercising boring.

With these partner cardio exercises, you get a level of interactivity that is missing on treadmills or exercise bikes and as a result they're a lot more fun.

1. Jogging On The Spot With A Partner

Equipment Required:
None.

Instructions:
Stand face to face with your partner and get them to crouch in front of you and raise their hands to your hip height. Start jogging on the spot and make sure your knees touch your partner's hands. Keep jogging for one minute.

Switch positions, crouch in front of your partner and raise your hands to their hip height. Get your partner to start jogging on the spot and make sure their knees touch your hands.

Get them to keep jogging for one minute. Repeat for as many repetitions as you desire.

Jogging On The Spot With A Partner Variations:
Jogging on the spot with a partner is a great way to burn some extra calories and boost your cardiovascular fitness. However, once your fitness levels improve, try the variation below to maximize the benefit you get from this exercise:

- *Jog on the spot for 10 seconds and then jump up in the air.*

- *Continue jogging and jumping in 10 second intervals and then swap with your partner every minute.*

- *Wear ankle and wrist weights while jogging on the spot with a partner to strengthen your muscles at the same time as boosting your cardiovascular fitness.*

2. Partner Burpees

Equipment Required:
1 small medicine ball.

Instructions:
Grab the medicine ball and stand about 10 feet away from your partner. Bend over, put the medicine ball on the floor, place your hands at either side of it and perform a burpee by kicking your legs out and then tucking them back in.

Grab the medicine ball, stand up straight and throw it to your partner. Get them to bend over, put the medicine ball on the floor and perform a burpee by kicking their legs out and tucking them back in.

Repeat for as many repetitions as you desire.

Partner Burpees Variations:
Partner burpees are a very challenging cardiovascular exercise. However, if you want to make them even tougher, give the following variations a try:

- *When you kick your legs out, perform a press up before tucking your legs back in. This will help build up your chest muscles as well as your cardiovascular fitness.*

- *Wear ankle and wrist weights while performing partner burpees to tone your muscles at the same time as boosting your cardiovascular fitness.*

3. Partner Jump Rope

Equipment Required:
1 jump rope.

Instructions:
Grab one end of the jump rope in each of your right hands and stand shoulder to shoulder, facing in opposite directions.

Start rotating the jump rope and jumping over it in unison. Repeat for as many repetitions as you desire.

Partner Jump Rope Variations:
Getting coordinated while performing the partner jump rope exercise does take some getting used to. However, once you've practiced it a few times, make it even more challenging by trying the alternatives below:

- *Change the direction you rotate the rope every five skips to test your reflexes as well as your cardiovascular fitness.*
- *Wear ankle and wrist weights while performing the partner jump rope exercise. This will help boost your strength as well as your cardiovascular fitness.*

4. Partner Resistance Sprints

Equipment Required:
1 towel.

Instructions:
Stand in front of your partner and get them to wrap the towel around your waist. Start sprinting as your partner attempts to pull you back with the towel.

Switch positions and wrap the towel around your partner's waist.
Get them to start sprinting as you attempt to pull them back with the towel. Repeat for as many repetitions as you desire.

Partner Resistance Sprints Variations:
Partner resistance sprints are a highly effective, multi-functional exercise that builds strength, power and cardiovascular fitness.

To make them even more difficult, try the variations below:

- *Instead of running forwards, perform partner resistance sprints face to face and run backwards. This will improve your balance and coordination along with your strength and cardiovascular fitness.*

- *Wear ankle and wrist weights while performing the partner resistance sprints. This will help boost your strength as well as your cardiovascular fitness.*

5. Partner Tennis Ball Shuffle

Equipment Required:
1 tennis ball.

Instructions:
Find a space where you can shuffle 20 steps to the side and pass a tennis ball without anyone blocking your path. Grab the tennis ball and stand face to face with your partner, making sure that you are about 10 feet apart.

Start shuffling from side to side and get your partner to do the same. As you shuffle, throw the tennis ball to your partner and get them to throw it back. Keep shuffling for as long as you desire.

Partner Tennis Ball Shuffle Variations:
The partner shuffle with tennis ball is a fantastic exercise that boosts your cardiovascular fitness and reflexes. However, once you have got used to the basic moves, five the following variations a try:

- *Jump as you throw the tennis ball to each other to make it even harder to catch and further improve your reflexes.*

- *Wear ankle and wrist weights while performing the partner tennis ball shuffle exercise. This will increase your strength while also testing your cardiovascular fitness and reflexes.*

Summary – Formulate a Plan With Your Partner

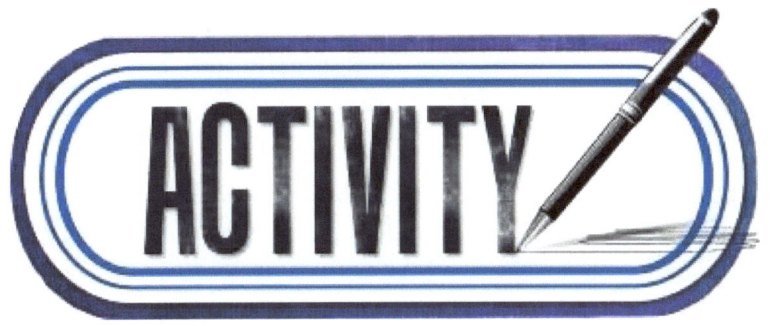

Working out with your partner is a great way to boost your fitness, strengthen your relationship and spend more quality time together. However, while learning about partner exercises is a good first step, to get the best results from these partner exercises, you need to formulate them into a solid workout plan.

To start formulating your workout plan, first decide which days and times you can both workout. Ideally, aim for 4-5 workouts each week but even if you can't fit that many workouts into your schedules, 1-2 workouts per week is better than nothing.

Once you've decided the days and times for your workout, you then need to decide which exercises you are going to be doing as part of each workout. To get the best results, you want to target the following areas at least once a week:

- *Biceps (Bic).*
- *Chest (Che).*
- *Cardio (Car).*
- *Core (Cor).*
- *Legs (Leg).*

- *Shoulders (Sho).*
- *Triceps (Tri).*
- *Upper Back (Bac).*

To make this a little easier, check out the matrix below that highlights which areas of the body each of the exercises listed in this eBook target:

	Bic	Che	Car	Cor	Leg	Sho	Tri	Bac
Partner Balance Exercises								
1. Back To Back Partner Stand Ups				✔	✔			
2. BOSU Tug Of War	✔			✔	✔	✔		✔
3. Single Leg Balance				✔	✔			
4. Single Leg BOSU Catch		✔		✔	✔	✔	✔	
5. Single Leg Partner Jump Shadow					✔			
Partner Bodyweight Exercises								
1. Bodyweight Partner Lunges	✔			✔	✔			✔
2. Bodyweight Partner Squats	✔			✔	✔			✔

	Bic	Che	Car	Cor	Leg	Sho	Tri	Bac
3. Partner Planks With Clap				✔				
4. Partner Push Ups With Clap		✔		✔		✔	✔	
5. Partner Wheelbarrow		✔		✔		✔	✔	
Partner Flexibility Exercises								
1. Back To Back Stretch					✔			✔
2. Partner Lying Hamstring Stretch					✔			
3. Partner Open Leg Stretch					✔			✔
4. Partner Shoulder Stretch						✔	✔	✔
5. Partner Tricep Stretch						✔	✔	✔
Partner Medicine Ball Exercises								
1. Medicine Ball Chest Pass		✔		✔	✔	✔	✔	

	Bic	Che	Car	Cor	Leg	Sho	Tri	Bac
2. Medicine Ball Partner Slams		✔			✔		✔	
3. Medicine Ball Partner Twists				✔				
4. Medicine Ball Sit Up & Pass				✔				
5. Medicine Ball Unders & Overs	✔	✔	✔	✔		✔	✔	✔
Partner Free Weight Exercises								
1. Negative Bicep Curls	✔							
2. Partner Barbell Deadlifts				✔	✔	✔		✔
3. Partner Barbell Sit Ups	✔			✔				
4. Partner Kettlebell Swings	✔			✔	✔	✔		
5. Superman Dumbbell Pass				✔		✔	✔	✔

	Bic	Che	Car	Cor	Leg	Sho	Tri	Bac
Partner Cardio Exercises								
1. Jogging On The Spot With A Partner			✔		✔			
2. Partner Burpees			✔	✔	✔			
3. Partner Jump Rope			✔		✔			
4. Partner Resistance Sprints			✔	✔	✔			
5. Partner Tennis Ball Shuffle			✔		✔			

Once you have all this information, you can then start to formulate your partner workout plan by picking at least five exercises per day. For example, a four-day partner workout program could look something like this:

- **Day 1 – Chest & Triceps (10 Minutes Per Exercise)** = Medicine Ball Chest Pass, Medicine Ball Partner Slams, Medicine Ball Sit Up & Pass, Partner Push Ups and Partner Wheelbarrows.
- **Day 2 – Upper Back & Biceps (10 Minutes Per Exercise)** = BOSU Tug Of War, Medicine Ball Unders & Overs, Negative Bicep Curls, Partner Kettlebell Swings and Superman Dumbbell Pass.

- **Day 3 – Legs & Shoulders (10 Minutes Per Exercise)** = Back To Back Partner Stand Ups, Bodyweight Partner Lunges, Bodyweight Partner Squats, Partner Shoulder Stretch and Single Leg BOSU Catch.
- **Day 4 – Core & Cardio (10 Minutes Per Exercise)** = Partner Barbell Deadlifts, Partner Barbell Sit Ups, Partner Burpees, Partner Jump Rope and Partner Tennis Ball Shuffle.

If you have more or less than four days, simply increase or decrease the areas you target each day. Then once the plan is completed, all that's left to do is start working out.

Good luck with your partner workout program!

Resources

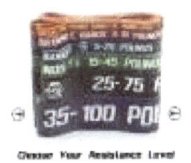

Resistance Bands - http://amzn.to/2p12hvG

BOSU Ball - http://amzn.to/2nK9wIr

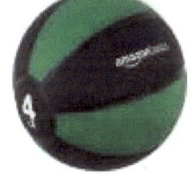

Medicine Ball - http://amzn.to/2oD61qR

Light Dumbbells - http://amzn.to/2o9KVzA

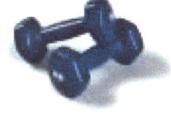

Wrist/Ankle Weights - http://amzn.to/2oD2clt

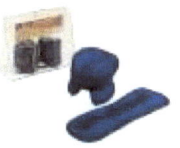

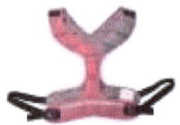 Weighted Vest - http://amzn.to/2nb6kJo

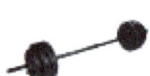 Barbell - http://amzn.to/2nEbLMq

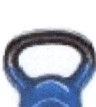 Kettlebell - http://amzn.to/2oDaSs5

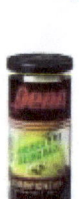 Tennis Ball - http://amzn.to/2nEcAoD

Other Relevant Books by This Author

If you would like to read more relevant books about this topic, here is a list of the CreateSpace links, titles and descriptions from this author:

https://www.createspace.com/6880021

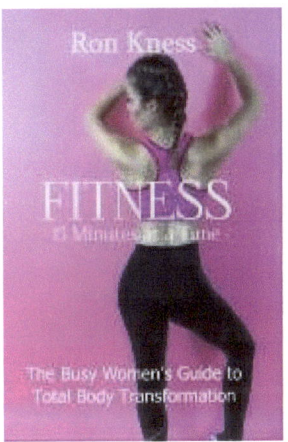

FITNESS - 15 Minutes at a Time: The Busy Women's Guide to Total Body Transformation

We want to be healthier. We also want to be empowered with maintaining our weight and fitness level. And we want to keep the weight off and maintain our healthy lifestyle for the rest of our life!

We can achieve ALL of these goals with the newest release from Ron Kness called "Fitness 15 Minutes at a Time". Based on these exciting teachings, you will learn about all the dramatic benefits of getting fit by eating healthy food resulting in weight loss, and doing high intensity exercising.

This book is built around a very clear, concept: improving your appearance and health.

It's not just about getting healthy. Having great fitness level is linked to reducing the risk of many diseases and even reversing the effects of some, such as being overweight and out of shape. These are just two of the many health benefits of being fit and at a normal weight.

In this book, we look at all the ways you can improve your own fitness level, starting with making the decision to get lose weight and healthy. That is the first step - you must want to do it!

This book also looks at the many other steps that can be taken to support this goal, from creating a calorie deficit - burning more calories than you eat - to exercising at a high intensity, to switching to a fitness and weight maintenance mode once at goal . The choices you make about the kind of food you eat and portion sizes has a big impact on your fitness level.

In "Fitness 15 Minutes at a Time", we'll cover all the bases, giving you everything you need to know to eat healthy, lose weight and get fit.

https://www.createspace.com/6988390

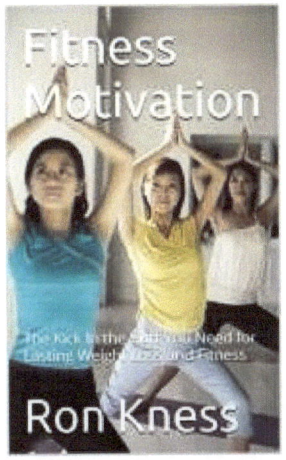

Fitness Motivation: The Kick In the Butt You Need for Lasting Weight Loss and Fitness

We want to be better about ourselves. We also want to be in control of our weight loss and fitness program. And we want to overcome adversity and negativity when on a weight loss and fitness program!

We can achieve ALL of these goals with the newest release from Ron Kness called "Fitness Motivation". Based on these exciting teachings, you will learn about all the dramatic benefits of staying the course when on a weight loss and fitness program and the immense value of having a positive mindset and eliminating negativity when trying to get fit.

This book is built around a very clear, concept: ultimately improve your body image through weight loss and fitness.

It's not just about learning to like yourself the way you are, although that can be hard in itself. Having great body image and high self-esteem is linked to being in charge of your own thinking. This is in part because you refuse to give in to body shaming and remove it from your life when possible.

In this book, we look at many different ways you can improve your own self-body image and self-esteem, starting with getting rid of negativity in your life. If that means dissolving some friendships that have a negative impact on you, then so be it!

This book will also look at the many other steps that can be taken to support this goal, from first determining what is causing adversity and negativity in your life to eliminating and replacing it with positivity. Even the choices you make about diet rewards and penalties can have an impact on your body image and self-esteem.

In "Fitness Motivation", we'll cover all the bases, giving you everything you need to know to stay motivated, learn from past failures, and to lose weight and get in great shape!

https://www.createspace.com/7038926

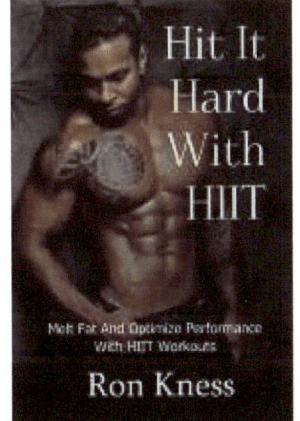

Hit It Hard With HIIT!: How to Melt Fat And Optimize Performance With High Intensity Interval Training (HIIT) Workouts

Think working out and getting in shape requires spending hours in the gym each day? It doesn't...

Discover how to quickly melt your extra fat, build muscle, and get in the best shape of your life with short workouts that take just minutes...

The fact is this...
You DON'T have to spend countless hours in the gym each week to get results.

Did you know that working out too much can actually slow down your results with working out?

It's true.

Over-exercising is one of the big reasons people struggle to get results and in some cases even end up injured from it.
- Forget about fad diets...
- Forget about long, grueling gym sessions...
- Forget about working out for hours each day...

If you're serious about melting fat, building muscle, and getting stronger faster than ever...

You need to focus on High Intensity Interval Training (HIIT)...

Here's why HIIT is superior to almost any weight loss or muscle-building program out there...
- Anyone can do it and get results regardless of current fitness levels
- You don't have to spend a crazy amount of time at the gym each day... you can do HIIT in just minutes per day
- Research shows us that results with HIIT are better than traditional exercise and fitness programs
- Not only is it fun and rewarding, you'll feel a lot better after your workouts and avoid overtraining
- You'll begin seeing noticeable results EXTREMELY quickly... forget about waiting weeks or months... most people start getting results in as little as a week or two (sometimes even days)

Here's what you'll discover inside...
- The old way of doing cardio training, why it's not all that effective, and how to do cardio the HIIT way for faster, better results...
- The science behind HIIT, why it's so powerful, and how to understand your own body to get the most out of it...
- The power of energy systems is revealed in detail inside and how we progress through energy systems for max results...

If you're starting from scratch and haven't worked out in a long time, you'll discover how to build a basic level of fitness...

Should you use machines in your HIIT training? The answer is revealed inside...
- How to maximize your results with kettlebells...

- The power of the "kettlebell swing" and how to do it the right way for amazing results...

- Advanced HIIT methods such as Tabata, cardio acceleration, Fartlek, and MetCon...

- Create whole-body circuit routines and the exact steps to design the PERFECT circuit routine...

- Why you may be working out too much and how to work out less and lose more fat and gain more muscle...

- And, how to incorporate HIIT with an overall healthy lifestyle...

- Plus, a whole lot more...

This is the ultimate step-by-step guide for using high intensity interval training to get into the best shape of your life.

Get Your HIIT Guide now (really, within minutes) and start getting in the best shape of your life tomorrow!

About the Author

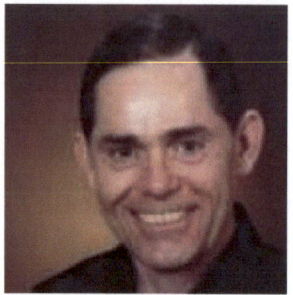

I have published over 125 books on Amazon for Kindle, CreateSpace and other publishing platforms.

While most of my books are on health and fitness in general, as I age (now 65) at the time of this writing) my topics of interest are geared toward aging baby boomers and older.

Besides my own writing, I also ghostwrite ebooks, books, reports, articles, blogs and do Kindle conversions for clients on a variety of topics.

Today my wife and I are retired from our careers and live in Gold Canyon, AZ. I now write as a retirement business where you'll find me happily sitting in my office typing away on my laptop as I work on my next book or ghostwriting project . . . that is if we are not traveling on a cruise ship - our new-found mode of travel.

www.ingramcontent.com/pod-product-compliance
Lightning Source LLC
Chambersburg PA
CBHW050817290526
45792CB00001B/155